THE Olive Leaf

Unequalled Immune Support for Health and Longevity

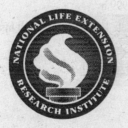

A Report from
The National Life Extension
Research Institute

The Olive Leaf:
Unequalled Immune Support for Health and Longevity

FIFTH PRINTING
Copyright © 1999 by
The National Life Extension Research Institute, Inc.
1675 E. Main Street, #221
Kent, Ohio 44240

All rights reserved. No part of this publication may be reproduced, stored in a retrieval system, or transmitted, in any form or by any means, electronic, mechanical, photocopying, recording, or otherwise, without the prior written permission of the publisher. Printed in the United States of America.

IMPORTANT:

The information herein is intended to help you make informed decisions about your diet and health, not to substitute for any treatment that may have been prescribed by your physician. If you suspect that you have a medical problem, we urge you to seek competent medical help. Keep in mind that nutritional needs vary from person to person, depending on age, sex, and total diet. Because there may be some individual risks involved, the publisher and researchers are not responsible for any adverse effects or consequences resulting from the use or misuse of any of the suggestions, preparations, or procedures in the Report.

These statements have not been evaluated by the Food and Drug Administration. The information is not intended to diagnose, treat, cure or prevent any disease but rather is intended solely for nutritional use. A testimonial reflects the personal experience of one person. Individual results may vary.

Table of Contents

Introduction

I'm sure you can remember where you were and what you were doing when:

...You first heard that President John F. Kennedy had been killed.

...Neil Armstrong took that "giant leap for mankind" and became the first man to walk on the moon.

...Richard Nixon went on national television and resigned the Presidency.

Take note of where you are and what you are doing right now.

While this event may not get the media coverage of these other momentous occasions, there is likely no other event in this decade, or the next, that will make such a profound personal difference in your life.

For this is the day that olive leaf extract frees all of us from fearing many of western society's most dreaded conditions of ill health.

But more importantly, olive leaf extract provides comfort, energy and the power for daily abundant living. Powerful health and a long, prosperous life can be ours.

Why, that sounds like the Tree of Life -- and so it just may be.

Robert Concoby
Director of Research
National Life Extension
Research Institute

Chapter 1

Olive Leaves: For the Health of the Nations

Scientists and those seeking the panacea for all of man's ills have often pondered the "Tree of Life" mentioned in the Bible. The 22nd chapter of Revelation states that:

> ...[T]he tree of life, which bare twelve manner of fruits, and yielded her fruit every month: and the leaves of the tree were for the healing of the nations.

Although it is unknown if such a tree is currently growing on the Earth, there is considerable historical, religious and scientific information relating to the olive tree that causes many to speculate.

The olive has the special biblical distinction of being the first herb named after the flood.

> *And the dove came in to him in the*
> *evening; and, lo, in her mouth was*
> *an olive leaf pluckt off: so Noah*
> *knew that the waters were abated*
> *from off the earth.*

GENESIS 8:11

Some believe that God may have been communicating something to Noah besides the fact that the earth was dry. In any event, Scripture has far more to say about the olive — its fruit, oil, wood — than any other tree.

Olive oil was part of the special ointment used to anoint priests and kings. Solomon crafted the two cherubim who were to guard the Ark of the Covenant in the Temple's Holiest Place from olive wood.

Christ often retreated to the Mount of Olives with his disciples to teach and pray. Some think that the very olive trees under which he prayed on the night before his passion are still alive and healthy today. In fact, the name of the Garden of Gethsemane comes from the Hebrew *Gatshamanim*, which literally translates as "oil press".[20]

Early Judeo-Christian legend holds that Adam, on his deathbed, asked for the oil of mercy which the Lord had given him for his own and all peoples' redemption. He

---

Table 1

Scientific Discoveries Concerning Olive Derivatives and Calcium Elenolate

Calcium elenolate has shown the ability to:

- Lower blood pressure in animals
- Increase blood circulation
- Help relieve certain heart problems
- Support the cardiovascular system
- Act effectively at low concentrations without harmful influence on cell mechanisms
- Be extremely safe and non-toxic, even at high amounts
- Lower 'bad' cholesterol levels

Calcium elenolate has been shown to have:

- a powerful anti-microbial action
- a killer effect against many viruses, bacteria and other microbes
- potency against a variety of viruses associated with the common ailments
- significant antioxidant activity against deadly free radicals

---

sent his son Seth to the angel that guarded the Garden of Eden. The angel gave Seth three seeds from the tree of knowledge, out of which grew a cedar, cypress and olive tree.

Perhaps this legend is one reason why, by the sixth century, it was a capital offense in Greece to kill or cut down an olive tree. [21] Also, at one time in Greece, only virgins or chaste young men were allowed to harvest the trees.[22]

When the Jews declared the miracle of Hanukkah because their eternal flame flickered eight days on empty, their fuel was olive oil.[22]

There are several other biblical references to olives, but it is sufficient to say that the olive occupies a special place in Jewish and Christian history.

Even before the first book of the Bible was ever penned, man revered the wonderful fruit of the olive tree and the oil produced from the fruit. Throughout history, the olive tree has inspired such notables as Vincent van Gogh and Renoir to paint and muse over their own olive trees with great reverence and awe.[22]

Today, the health benefits of olive oil continue to be extolled by both herbalists and medical science.

Greer and Blau mention the lowering of cholesterol levels, increased circulation, gastric healing, the removing of gallstones and the prevention of diabetes and atherosclerosis as being associated with increased olive oil consumption, as well as the oil's natural antioxidant capabilities.[20]

Ancient Egyptians revered the olive leaf, and used olive oil to mummify the pharaohs. Modern science is still discovering the unexplainable preservation abilities of olive products, especially the olive leaf.

Throughout earlier ages, tea made from olive leaves has been a popular folk remedy for combating fevers.

Medical reports from as early as 1827 report that a tea made from olive leaves helped the worst cases of malaria. It was found to be far superior to quinine, the recommended treatment of the time. A doctor from that time believed that a bitter substance in the olive leaf was responsible for its potent healing power.

Early in this century, the bitter compound was isolated from the olive leaf. This phytochemical, called oleuropein, provides the olive tree with vast disease-resistant properties.

Oleuropein is credited with the olive tree's ability to live for thousands of years — it protects the tree against nearly every disease.

Elenolic Acid — the "miracle" ingredient

In 1969, scientists in the Department of Virology Research at The Upjohn Company in Michigan isolated even more active compounds from olive leaves — elenolates — that kill microbes.   In the body, oleuropein is hydrolized into elenolic acid. Upjohn performed their studies on a salt of elenolic acid called calcium elenolate.

Since that time, they have been studying the effect of these extractions from the olive leaf. Many of these studies will be referenced later in this book but some of their findings are summarized in Table 1-1 above.

The properties of calcium elenolate so encouraged the people at Upjohn that they spent much time and money in an attempt to synthesize and patent a "miracle" antibiotic. They discovered a problem that they were unable to overcome.

Although calcium elenolate showed unequaled therapeutic effects in vitro (in a test tube) it was discovered that it was only effective in vivo (in the body) for a few minutes. They determined that calcium elenolate binds to amino acids in the blood stream thus inactivating its anti-microbial properties.

Elenolic acid, not calcium elenolate, is produced in the body as oleuropein comes in contact with certain enzymes present in the bloodstream of all warm blooded mammals.

The researchers at Upjohn chose to restrict their focus to calcium elenolate, and ran into the problem stated above. Unable to overcome this problem using calcium elenolate only, and not elenolic acid, they abandoned the project and gave up on their research.

Several years ago independent scientific research produced the breakthrough that opened the way for application of a natural olive leaf extract product. Not focusing on calcium elenolate as Upjohn did, these researchers chose to spend their time and attention on elenolic acid, which yielded an important scientific breakthrough.

Chapter 2

The Vital
Scientific Breakthrough

In 1969, the promises of olive leaf extract for vibrant health aroused the interest of the medical community.

Upjohn found that one of the ingredients in olive leaf extract, calcium elenolate, destroyed every harmful virus, bacteria, yeast, fungi and protozoan it was exposed to invitro (in the test tube).

Unfortunately, they also discovered that calcium elenolate binds to amino acids in vivo (in the body), and thus becomes inactive within minutes.

As mentioned previously, the nutriceutical actually responsible for the pathogenic properties of olive leaf extract is elenolic acid, produced in the bloodstream by the exposure of oleuropein to certain enzymes.

Two Forms of Elenolic Acid

Further research determined that there are two forms of elenolates, *l*-elenolates and *d*-elenolates, produced by the olive leaf. Biochemists call these two forms stereo isomers. The best way to understand stereo isomers is to look at human hands.

Each hand has four fingers and a thumb. Both hands are similar except in the way the fingers and thumb are configured on the hand. In like manner, the two stereo isomers of elenolate have the same chemical composition but are strung together so that one is the mirror image of the other.

Many organic compounds have stereo isomers. Most amino acids have left and right handed molecules. For example, if one looks on the ingredient listing of a protein supplement, one will see *l*-arginine and *l*-carnitine. The "*l*" signifies the left handed molecule.

Nature also produces an equal amount of *d*-arginine and *d*-carnitine but the designer of life chose only to use left-handed amino acids to make DNA, RNA and other proteins. The "*d*" is scientific shorthand for right-handed molecules.

In like manner, the designer has chosen the right handed elenolate molecule, *d*-elenolate, to be of value against microorganisms.

The way scientists determine whether a molecule is left-handed or right-handed is in the way the molecule reflects polarized light. *l*-elenolate molecules reflect polarized light to the left and *d*-elenolate molecules reflect to the right.

The Final Breakthrough

Using the previous biochemical research as a starting point, other researchers began to look for the secret of developing an olive leaf extract that works in the body for longer than a few minutes.

Working tirelessly for more than six years, one company spent hundreds of thousands of dollars. In 1995, they discovered the solution to the mystery. They have now obtained patent protection for their proprietary extraction process. That process results in a concentration of right-reflecting

molecules of elenolic acid in the body, in a
natural olive leaf product.

Chapter 3

How does Olive Leaf Extract Work?

Immune System Support

Humans have an elaborate immune system. That system acts as a coat of armor to protect us from the billions of pathogenic (disease-causing) organisms in our environment and that enter the body through breathing, eating, drinking and cuts in the skin.

When the immune system is functioning at the peak of efficiency, these microorganisms can be present in ones' body but they have little effect. However, when an injury or an over abundance of physical or mental stress weakens the immune system, these opportunistic germs are able to get a stronghold.

Disease results as these pathogens overtake various glands, organs and tissues in the body. At some point, the diseased glands, organs or tissues produce symptoms that are characteristic of the particular pathogen. For example, cold viruses normally attack the respiratory system. The respiratory system then reacts by producing more phlegm. Tissues swell, then sneezing, coughing, runny nose, and other discomforts appear as symptoms.

Sometimes the symptoms are immediate. But, many times it takes months and even years for them to appear. Even prior to the appearance of symptoms, the pathogens are in the body draining strength from the infected tissues and the immune system.

The ingredients in olive leaf extract support and boost the immune system.

Olive Leaf Extract is Not a Drug

It is also important to realize that olive leaf extract is not a drug. As a result, taken in recommended amounts, one may not notice an overnight improvement. In some cases of serious immune system problems, two or three months of regular ingestion are required before significant improvements in chronic conditions of ill health are realized.

IMPORTANT: Olive Leaf Extract IS NOT a Cure

Olive leaf extract does not cure disease. It is important to remember that pathogens are not the disease. Neither are symptoms the disease. Disease occurs as pathogens or other harmful substances damage glands, organs or tissues of the body.

Nothing in the extract can change or fix damaged cells in the body.

By attacking microbes and directly strengthening the body's immune system, olive leaf extract enables the immune system to better protect and help restore health.

Olive leaf extract can simply help improve and maintain the immune system and healthy body function.

Chapter 4

The Detox Effect:

a Good Sign

In some cases where people are suffering with a chronic problem, there may be a quick and somewhat adverse reaction, called a Herxheimer Reaction.[29]

Commonly called detox, this refers to symptoms generated by a detoxification process.

As the body begins to deal with dead microbes, one may experience a variety of detox symptoms.

This occurs as invading organisms die. Dead microbes may be present throughout the body. When large quantities of dead microbes are present, the body begins a process to get rid of them.

Sometimes it's more than the eliminative organs can handle at one time. The liver, kidneys, intestines and skin may become over-burdened. Thus, one could feel ill or develop a skin reaction. All of these conditions are good signs — they indicate that the olive leaf extract is working to help the body combat germs that may be causing various conditions of ill health.

Common reactions include fatigue, diarrhea, headaches, muscle/joint achiness or flu-like symptoms. Some people may develop a rash, pimples or other skin condition. Severity differs also from person to person, depending on the extent of the problem.

How To Handle Detox Effect

The best way to maximize the power of olive leaf extract and limit any adverse reaction is to *drink four cups of water in between usages*. Water helps to strengthen the lymphatic system and flush the kidneys.

In the event substantial detoxification symptoms occur that produce discomfort, the first line of attack is to drink a large amount of distilled or reverse osmosis water. If detox symptoms persist, there are other courses of action as well.

For minimal discomfort, such as a headache or muscle/joint pain, a simple over-the-counter analgesic such as aspirin or ibuprofen usually suffices.

For more than minimal discomfort, one might consider reducing the daily intake of olive leaf extract. One might even stop taking it altogether for a few days. It may take a short time for the body to eliminate the toxins and dead microbes.

After these few days, one should resume taking olive leaf extract at a lower amount and increase slowly.

Safety Studies with Olive Leaf Extract

Research indicates that amounts many times higher than recommended are unlikely to produce toxic or other adverse side effects.[1] During 1993 testing of an early liquid form of olive leaf extract, there were no observed or reported side effects.

Die-off effect is only temporary. In spite of the detoxification effect in some individuals, olive leaf extract is very safe.

Chapter 5

Olive Leaf Extract and Increased Energy

Olive leaf extract produces substantial energy increases in most people that use it. It is not at all uncommon to hear people state that they have more energy than they have had for years.

One likely reason for this is that the body is now freed from fighting so many opportunistic invaders. Without having to direct much of its energy inward for immune processes, the body can redirect that energy level outwards to be used as desired.

One frequently heard comment is that most people have more energy and feel more alive. Healthy people without any noticeable health problems who take it say they also feel this infusion of energy.

Chapter 6

Beating Debilitating Fatigue

Chronic Fatigue Syndrome is a rather prevalent condition of late. While it may seem like a rather new problem, Chronic Fatigue Syndrome is related to the more widely known malady, mononucleosis, commonly called the "kissing disease" years ago, a reference to the method of transmission.

Viral Origin of Chronic Fatigue

Both mononucleosis and Chronic Fatigue Syndrome (myalgic encephalo-myelitis) are caused by the same virus. This virus is a member of the herpes family, and is related to the viruses that cause shingles (herpes zoster), chickenpox, glandular fever, herpes simplex I&II, and cytomegalo-

virus.[25,30] Both mononucleosis and chronic
fatigue are caused by the Epstein-Barr virus.

Since sufferers of Chronic Fatigue
Syndrome also exhibit weakened immune
systems, the acronym CFIDS, short for
Chronic Fatigue Immune Dysfunction
Syndrome, is used to describe the condi-
tion.[31]

The symptoms of CFIDS include, of
course, bone-crushing fatigue as well as
fever, sore throat, swollen glands, allergies,
insomnia or hypersomnia, frequent colds or
infections, menstrual problems or PMS, low
blood sugar (hypoglycemia), anemia, indigestion or other digestive problems, depression, memory loss, loss of concentration,
anxiety, stress, headache and other aches and
pains.

HSV/Epstein-Barr Infection Lasts for a Lifetime

After the virus enters the body via a
primary infection, it then travels up the
nerve to a cluster of cells known as the nerve
ganglion. There it remains, hiding from the
immune system, waiting to move to the
skin's surface and reinfect at a later time,

usually after a period of undue stress, immune system compromise, old age, disease or drug or alcohol use.[30]

Virtually all Adults Infected with Epstein-Barr

The herpes family of viruses (HSV) or Epstein-Barr (EBV) afflicts most people before or shortly upon reaching adulthood. Blood studies done on people living in cities have shown that 95% of adults test positive for some previous infection with HSV.[26] Stoff and Pellegrino state that virtually everyone is infected with the Epstein-Barr virus, and that it can live in one's body for 60 years or longer.[30]

In the elderly population, herpes infection is even more pronounced. Nearly 100% of the elderly test positive for herpes antibodies, indicating a previous infection.[27] Drs. Stoff and Pellegrino estimate that by the first year of college, up to 80% of adults are or have been infected with EBV, and the number continues to increase yearly until by age 30, 97% of adults test positive for EBV infection.[30]

A dangerous scenario develops when a herpes infection spreads to the brain as encephalitis or meningitis. Normal flu symptoms occur at the beginning, sometimes followed by paralysis, hallucinations and other serious behavior disturbances. Blindness, deafness or even death can result.[25,30]

Chronic Epstein-Barr virus can also lead to autoimmune diseases such as lupus, nerve pain, numbness, seizures or paralysis. These are very serious illnesses, and must not be taken lightly. Proper medical attention is needed immediately.

Of even more disturbing news is the data that some researchers are now discovering. The instances of infection has been doubling since 1984. They believe that Epstein-Barr has either changed and mutated, or that a new and different virus infects a person, which awakens the dormant Epstein-Barr. This has become a serious problem. The likely suspect for this viral epidemic: human B-lymphotropic virus, HBLV, also called human herpes virus 6.[30]

Some medical doctors and researchers surmise that there is a connection between the Epstein-Barr virus and a particular form of cancer called nasopharyngeal carcinoma. This cancer is approaching an epidemic proportion in China, where young children routinely contract the Epstein-Barr virus.[30]

Since Epstein-Barr is a virus, no antibiotic has any power against it. The same frightening scenario exists for the other viruses mentioned above.

Esptein-Barr can also lead to various secondary infections, such as strep throat from streptococcus.

Olive Leaf Extract - A Potent Protector

All of this would paint a rather bleak picture, were it not for the existence of olive leaf extract. A good number of people have reported the elimination of fatigue-type problems after using olive leaf extract.

Laboratory testing demonstrates that olive leaf extract kills various viruses, both in vitro and in vivo. See the charts in the Appendices for a more complete listing.

Fibromyalgia

Fibromyalgia is another syndrome that has been diagnosed with increasing frequency over the last few years, much like Chronic Fatigue Syndrome.

Approximately 2.5% of the total population has fibromyalgia, while up to 20% or more of the female population between the ages of 40 and 60 years old have the symptoms. Of great interest is that the syndrome occurs most frequently in the under-40 year old age group.

Simply defined, fibromyalgia is an unusual disorder that manifests itself in various parts of the body. In the early days of this new syndrome, many practitioners simply called any soft tissue-type problem that they couldn't otherwise diagnose as fibromyalgia.

Today, diagnosis is much more specific. The symptoms of fibromyalgia include aches, pains, stiffness, localized tenderness and swelling, fatigue, stress, headache, sore throat, intestinal problems, depression, anxiety, memory blanks, loss of concentration, mood swings and fitful sleep.

Fibromyalgia and CFIDS Linked

Note the substantial similarity in symptoms of fibromyalgia with those of Chronic Fatigue Syndrome. There have been some immunologic antibody findings that indicate a pathogenic-linked cause for fibromyalgia, just like Chronic Fatigue Syndrome. Many researchers today link fibromyalgia in some manner with CFIDS. Dr. Walter Gunn states "What seems to show up in article after article is some kind of immune dysfunction." Whether these abnormalities are due to a viral infection, a reactivation of latent viruses or another factor is as yet unproven. It is known however, that a large number of infectious agents initiate the onset of fibromyalgia.[3]

Additionally, two different laboratories have found that fibromyalgia is accompanied by low levels of natural killer cell activity.[3] Olive leaf extract empowers the immune system by increasing the body's ability to produce white blood cells, the body's natural killer cells.

Olive leaf extract also has a proven record in vitro against both viruses as well as numerous other pathogens.

Chapter 7

Olive Leaf Extract
and the Heart

It is now well-known and well documented that one product of the olive tree, olive oil, has a positive health benefit to the cardiovascular system. The Mediterranean Diet, of which olive oil is a part, is beneficial when used as part of a healthy lifestyle. It must also be remembered that olive oil is rich in various olive phenolics which likely accounts for much of its nutritional power.

Petroni and Blasevich at the Institute of Pharmacological Studies, University of Milan found that a phenol-enriched olive oil extract reduced blood platelet aggregation.

As reported in the April, 1995 issue of Thrombosis Research, they determined that this beneficial effect was caused by the antioxidant properties in the extra-virgin olive oil. Of equal, or perhaps even more importance, they also found that the aqueous waste water from the olive oil refining process, rich in phenolics, showed rather potent activities as well. Oleuropein, luteolin, apigenin and quercetin were less active than the phenol-enriched extract.[4]

Serious cardiovascular system problems

Petroni and Blasevich's partners at the University of Milan, F. Visioli and C. Galli, paved the way in their 1994 study which showed that olive derivatives are good antioxidants. Thus, they proposed that the Mediterranean diet helps prevent some heart problems.[5]

V. Petkov, working on his research in Europe and writing for peer-review journals, also found uses for olive derivatives in nutritionally maintaining healthy cardiovascular systems.[6]

Low Density Lipids and Cholesterol

Perez-Jimenez and Espino, in their 1995 article in the American Journal of Clinical Nutrition, demonstrated that a diet rich in olive oil increased the high-density lipids, or good cholesterol, by 7%.[7]

A 1994 experiment at the University of Milan's Institute of Pharmacological Sciences found that oleuropein inhibited oxidation of low-density lipoproteins, the so-called "bad cholesterol" connected to various heart problems.[5]

A subsequent study in 1995 at the same institution linked olive constituents to the reduction or delaying of problems in the heart.[8]

The 1996 study by Ruiz-Guttierrez and Muriana at the University Hospital found that components in olive oil significantly boosted high-density lipids ("good" cholesterol) and reduced the low-density lipids ("bad" cholesterol).[9]

Olive Leaf Maintains Proper Blood Pressure

Olive leaf extract has also been studied for its ability to lower blood pressure. Ribeiro and Fiuza reported the findings of their study in the Journal of Ethnopharmacology. They studied thirty two medicinal plants, and verified that olea europaea, olive leaf, produced a beneficial effect.[10]

These findings were confirmed by A. Zarzuelo and J. Duarte, researchers in the Pharmacology Department at the University of Granada, Spain, who studied olive leaf. They showed that oleuropein is largely responsible for this good effect, but that there was also one other compound in the olive leaf that potentiates this pressure-lessening action.[11]

A recent study of olive leaf to determine its blood pressure lowering capabilities was undertaken in 1996 by a large team of researchers in Belgium. They tested thirty patients who were suffering from high blood pressure. After three months on olive leaf extract, all thirty patients experienced a decrease in blood pressure. Quoting the researchers, "We note for all patients a statistically significant decrease of blood pressure." Additionally, they noted that they did not find any side effects from the olive leaf extract occurring in the patients in this study.[12]

Another 1996 study from the University Hospital in Sevilla, Spain found that phenolic-rich olive oil reduced both the systolic and diastolic blood pressures.[9]

As demonstrated here, olive leaf extract is a powerful antioxidant much like flavonoids and proanthocyanidins. These very compounds protect the heart and cardiovascular system from free radical-induced damage, and promote powerful good health in the user.

Chapter 8

Olive Leaf Extract, Colds and Flu

Eighty years ago, a killer flu killed 21 million people worldwide. It left pain, suffering, death and broken families in its wake. The mortality rate was 10 times worse than the normal strain of influenza. This new flu strain caught the world by surprise.

Many people had fevers of 104 degrees, and died as their lungs filled with fluid. Many became delirious before they died. In the U.S., 675,000 people died from the flu in less than a year's time. Its impact worldwide was worse than Europe's black plague of the Middle Ages.

This killer flu was called the Spanish flu, believing that it had originated in Spain. That was incorrect — most likely, the killer flu of 1918 originated in China, where most new flu strains are born.[13]

Which gives one pause, considering that in late 1997, Hong Kong panicked upon discovery of an avian influenza, aptly named the "bird flu." A flu strain previously limited to birds appeared in humans, and afflicted a number of people. Authorities worried that the virus might mutate into a form more easily passed among humans. Authorities killed more than one million birds in hopes of eliminating the disease carriers.

While it appears that the disease was halted, one scientist remained wary. He's quoted as saying "It's a lull in the battle. We can't say it's still not lurking somewhere."[13]

While these events are certainly scary, one need not excessively fear health problems caused by flu, colds, or their related problems, such as pneumonia, in the case of influenza.

Almost Half the U.S. Population Suffers Every Year

Many Americans fall prey to several colds every year. Additionally, in 1990, 43.4% of Americans suffered through at least one bout of the flu. That's more than

100 million people missing work, school and other important aspects of their lives due to a virus. Anecdotally, the single largest cause of missed work or school are viral cold and flu infections.

Laboratory testing shows that olive leaf extract could substantially reduce one's susceptibility to cold or flu viruses. (Turn to the Appendix for listings of the many pathogens that olive leaf extract counters in vitro.)

In a meeting with Dr. Robert Lyons, O.M.D. in August, 1998, he stated that he has a very high success rate using olive leaf extract against various viral problems. He further stated that he is personally unafraid of almost any pathogen that he might be exposed to due to his strong belief in the power of olive leaf extract.

Olive leaf extract appears to offer organic health benefits not available with pharmaceutical antibiotics. Many people who lead stressful lives or who may be particularly susceptible to colds and viruses may benefit from long-term use of olive leaf extract as an immune system booster.

M.G. Soret, writing in Antimicrobial Agents and Chemotherapy, tested calcium elenolate against the parainfluenza 3 virus. He found that it was virucidal when given within minutes of exposure to the virus. He found that, when given at 2 or 3 hours before exposure, as well as at 18 hours after exposure, calcium elenolate had no antiviral effect.

The parainfluenza 3 virus was inhibited when calcium elenolate was given either 15 minutes before or after exposure. Decreasing the time from 15 minutes to 10 or 5 minutes before and after exposure "increased the effectiveness of calcium elenolate."[35]

Chapter 9

Immunity and Antibiotics in Crisis

The human immune system is an incredibly complicated design. Beginning with the skin, this tough barrier stops most pathogens from entering our bodies. But for those that do get through, an army of killer cells awaits the hapless germ.

As microbes enter our bodies, our immune system recognizes them as proteins that are different from the normal ones found in our bodies. The inflammatory response moves into action, surrounding the invader with phagocytes, white blood cells. To do this, the body widens the blood vessels in the affected area. Swelling occurs, which is actually a good sign that the immune system is working.

Antibodies are then produced from B-lymphocyte cells which attach themselves to

the invading pathogen. These B-lympho-
cytes act as locator beacons for phagocytes,
which come and destroy the pathogen.

T-lymphocytes then spring into action,
latching on to cells that have been invaded
by the pathogen and killing them.

The Problem with Traditional Antibiotics

Our traditional treatment-of-choice
against infections has been various kinds of
antibiotics. We know that the mechanism by
which antibiotics work is perhaps not the
most beneficial to the human body. Many
antibiotics suppress the immune system, and
nearly all of them destroy beneficial organisms in the intestinal tract.[30]

Additionally, medical science has stated numerous times over recent years that the
current antibiotics have largely been ren-
dered of little use against the newly-named
"superbug" germs. With no new antibiotics
on the horizon, this poses a grave threat to
health.[14]

It must be noted that this is a major
medical problem today of epidemic propor-
tions. Largely as a result of overuse of

antibiotics, many microbes are resistant to those medicines.

Today, there are few effective antibiotics available that continue to work with the most common pathogens. Some of the new strains of "superbugs" are totally unaffected by traditional drugs.

Olive Leaf Extract and the "Superbugs"

A series of testing with olive leaf extract shows a very interesting and immensely significant development. Olive leaf extract contains components called iridoids that create a structurally-complicated molecule. It appears that harmful microorganisms cannot readily develop a resistance to olive leaf extract's complex structure.

Incidentally, olive leaf extract does all this while enhancing immune system function, and leaving intact the beneficial bacteria in the intestines.

Tassou and Nychas, researchers at the Ministry of Agriculture in Athens, Greece detailed the results of their studies in the prestigious journals Lancet and Biotechnology and Applied Biochemistry stating that olive extract and oleuropein inhibits the germination and growth of the Bacillus cereus pathogen.[15]

Olive Leaf Extract Beats Germs

It is known that hospitals harbor some of the more virulent strains of microbes. This poses additional problems for the patient whose immune system is already overburdened or compromised.

Up to 40% of the people in a community may carry staph colonies, while up to 70% of people in hospitals have the bacteria.[23]

A common infector, Streptococcus pneumoniae are largely resistant to antibiotics. Parents take note that S. pneumoniae is a major cause of ear infections.[23]

Olive Leaf Extract Powerful and Safe against "Super Bugs."

Tranter and Tassou, of the PHLS Centre for Applied Microbiology and Research in England, found in 1993 that oleuropein inhibited the growth of Staphylococcus aureus when tested in vitro. A concentration of only 0.4-0.6% was sufficient for this anti-bacterial effect. A 0.1% concentration delayed but did not prevent growth. A 0.2% concentration inhibited growth in only one of two test media. They also noted that oleuropein was effective in the destruction of enterotoxin B.[16]

Olive leaf extract has also been tested and found to be safe in amounts far higher than the normal daily amount. Scientific testing indicates that amounts many times larger than the daily recommended usage are not toxic and do not cause adverse side effects.[1]

Garrido-Fernandez and Vaughn, reporting in the Canadian Journal of Microbiology, noted that oleuropein can possess antibacterial action, although the mechanism by which it works needs further study. They proposed that its antibacterial action was somehow related to carbon utilization. They found that a 0.2-0.4% concentration delayed the growth of some lactic acid bacteria, but had little effect on spoilage organisms.[33]

Capasso and Evidente, along with their team of 4 other researchers, found in 1995 that olive oil vegetation waters were highly toxic to a number of different bacterium. They tested it against Pseudomonas syringae, Pv. savastanoi (Gram-negative) and Corynebacterium michiganese (Gram-positive).[17]

Fleming, Walter and Etchells found that oleuropein did not inhibit lactic acid bacteria, but that two by-products, aglycone and elenolic acid, inhibited the four species of lactic acid bacteria tested. They did note that a crude oleuropein extract had an effect on only 3 of 17 species of non-lactic acid bacteria, while its acid hydrolosate inhibited 11 of the 17 bacteria.[34]

Chapter 10

Olive Leaf Extract and Parasites

Olive Leaf Extract Kills Parasites

Parasites are notoriously difficult to kill and expel from the body. Olive leaf extract exhibits promising anti-parasitic action against just such invaders.

Note: During a parasite cleanse, some people may become nauseated or experience other unpleasant feelings. This is most likely due to severe parasitic infection and the resultant "die-off" which releases toxins or dead parasites into the bloodstream.

Tropical Illnesses

Olive leaf extract offers considerable potential against malaria. Malaria is carried by infected mosquitoes which inject the parasite into the human as they inject their hypodermic tongue and withdraw blood.

The malaria protozoan views the human as another host to infect, and travels down the mosquito's tongue and into the body.[23]

It is reported that the Inca indians used quinine for malaria as early as the mid-seventeenth century.[23]

Beginning in the mid-nineteenth century, teas made with olive leaves were used with good success to fight malaria, and presumably other types of tropical illnesses as well. Today, olive leaf extract is a much easier and more convenient method of obtaining relief from these serious tropical problems.

Chapter 11

Olive Leaf Extract and Food Poisoning

Mortimer and McCann, English researchers writing a report in the May 1974 issue of Lancet, a prestigious medical journal, found that fried rice, a Chinese dish, was sometimes contaminated with the bacillus cereus bacteria.[18]

The poisoning brought on by bacillus cereus includes such symptoms as nausea, vomiting, diarrhea, and abdominal pain.

Researchers at the Athens Institute of Food Technology demonstrated that olive leaf extract effectively stops the outgrowth of B. cereus, and inhibits spread of the bacteria.

Researchers detailing the results of these studies in the prestigious journals Lancet and Biotechnology and Applied

Biochemistry report that oleuropein inhibited growth of Bacillus cereus T spores.[15]

Tassou and Nychas, reporting in the February 1995 issue of Letters in Applied Microbiology determined that the olive leaf extract phenolic oleuropein inhibited the growth of salmonella. There was no such inhibition in the control sample. They did note, however, that the inhibition caused by oleuropein was more pronounced at a low pH and low inoculum size.[19]

Chapter 12

Candida, Yeast and Fungal Problems

Candida albicans is a specific yeast which exists in a certain amount in the human body. It is found in the intestines, in the mouth, on the skin and throughout the digestive tract.

Normally it causes no problems, unless some change causes a supression of the immune system. It is in these situations, especially if the yeast is allowed to flourish and grow beyond a certain amount, that a situation called yeast overgrowth occurs. In this situation, the yeast overgrowth may result in a deep-seated infection, many times lodging in mucous membranes, the skin or nails.

In fact, systemic candida has become a common, life-threatening illness in weak or immune-suppressed individuals.[24] Some

health practitioners believe candida overgrowth to be a large problem today, especially in the western world. It must be noted
that candida albicans is a very different yeast
from that found in bread and foodstuffs.

It has only been since the 1960s that
candida albicans was found to be involved in
many chronic and systemic problems. Dr. C.
Orian Truss of Birmingham, Alabama was
the first to connect candida overgrowth with
various medical conditions. He followed his
thesis for several years, first reporting on his
findings at a medical conference in Toronto
in 1977, and publishing his data beginning in
1978.[28]

In very recent times, both in the western world and developing countries, there
has been a significant and dramatic increase
in the number of fungal and other microbial
infections. Richardson and Warnock estimate that up to 10% of all bloodstream
infections and 25% of all urinary tract infections in hospital settings are caused by yeast
organisms.[24]

It is estimated that up to 50% of the
adult population may have measureable

yeast overgrowth. Much higher rates of infection have been seen in persons seeking medical attention for various problems.

As shall be shown, modern laboratory methods for detecting these invaders have lagged behind and not kept pace with this epidemic onslaught. Only three species of fungus can readily be determined via blood cultures — the *candida* species, *Cryptococcus neoformans* or the *Trichosporon* species.[24]

Oral candida, commonly called thrush, afflicts many newborn infants during or shortly after birth. Many times, this is a result of the mother's vaginal candidosis, which afflicts 20% of the women population, on average. Another likely exposure to the infection is from the hands of the parents or hospital staff, since C. albicans can live on exposed skin tissues.[24]

Problems of Candidosis

Laboratory testing is of little use to determine a yeast overgrowth problem. As already mentioned, only three of multiple forms of fungus can be detected via a normal blood workup.

Various problems can be considered an indicator of candida albicans overgrowth (chronic candidiasis). These can be:

Fatigue, asthma, depression, headaches, muscle aches or weakness, joint pain, gastritis, constipation, diarrhea, gas, bloating, vaginal burning, itching or discharge, urinary tract problems, scalp and facial hair problems, prostatitis, jock itch, infertility, menstrual problems, PMS, allergies, mouth sores, nail infections, psoriasis, food allergies, itching, irritability, inability to concentrate, memory loss, skin problems, recurrent yeast infections or vaginitis in women, allergies and sugar cravings.

Causes of Yeast Overgrowth

Poor diets, especially those high in carbohydrates, sugar, yeast and yeast products, as well as molds and fermented foods provide a ripe breeding ground for candida.

Additionally, repeated exposure to antibiotics also pose a threat. For women, taking birth control pills or having multiple

---

Table 2

Possible Symptoms of a
Yeast Problem

- General sick feeling
- Fatigue & tiredness
- Headache
- Antibiotic use in past
- Hard to concentrate and remember things
- Joint pain
- Muscle aches or pain
- Allergies
- Digestion problems (bloating, gas, etc.)
- Premenstrual tension
- Cold hands or feet
- Sinus problems
- Skin problems
- Vaginitis (for women)
- Prostatitis (for men)

---

pregnancies can provide a favorable environment for growth of candida.

The overuse of antibiotics is a widely known fact today.

Removing the Yeast Overgrowth

In the past, various protocols have been used for candida elimination. Prescriptions of nystatin, a yeast-specific antibiotic are common. In numerous people, however, nystatin causes an allergic-type response.

A very restrictive candida diet is almost always prescribed as well. This diet virtually eliminates all yeast-containing or yeast-benefiting products from the diet, such as bread, cereal, wheat, potato, flour, coffee, herbs, honey, chocolate, ice cream, jelly, cheese, ketchup, mustard, pastries, bacon, sausage, vinegar, fermented foods, juices and the like.

Suffice it to say that such protocols are inconvenient and difficult to maintain.

Olive leaf extract produces beneficial results against various yeast problems while being much easier to use, and without any side effects.

Refer to Chapter 4 for more information on possible reactions and the "die-off" effect.

Chapter 13

Anecdotal Reports

IMPORTANT NOTE: Anecdotal reports are not valid for making scientific or categorical statements about the efficacy of any substance. These accounts have been taken from unsolicited letters on file from people who have used olive leaf extract.

Parasitic Problems

A woman suffering from malaria sought medical help. She exhibited the usual symptoms - yellow fingernails and ears, mucous discoloration, weight loss, tremors and anemic disposition. She began taking olive leaf extract and was completely rid of symptoms, as evidenced by 3 different laboratory tests of her blood.

Martha S., Mexico

Increased Energy/Musculoskeletal Problems

"I have been using olive leaf extract for one month. Results that I have noticed are my blood sugar is stable and have been able to maintain.   Energy has been great.   Also my wife has arthritis and has had to take medications but tried the olive leaf and found good results."   *Manuel G.*

Increased Energy

"I would strongly like to recommend olive leaf extract, which I took for one month. For the last few years I have not been feeling like myself. I've had little energy and enthusiasm for anything. This is not my usual nature. I attributed it to weight, unemployment and just being down. My head was always somewhat achy and I couldn't figure out why. The only way I could describe it would be as a constant low-degree headache which never left. I started taking olive leaf extract and noticed an immediate elevation of my spirits. What I liked about the product was that it was effective but gentle and didn't make me hyper or unable to sleep. Quite the contrary, I slept better. After a few days I began to notice more energy and a stronger sense of well-being. The cobwebs in my brain started to diminish. I also noticed a bad shoulder and a bad knee start to get better. The pain associated with these joints remarkably improved. This is a fabulous product. The only side effects I had were a couple of headaches in the beginning which disappeared with some aspirin. I started to feel much better. It was amazing to see the fatigue disappear and my general health improve. I couldn't believe I felt so well. This is an incredible product in that it actually reduces symptoms over a short period of time and fixes the problem. I stopped taking olive leaf extract after 30 days and experienced no withdrawal or anything. I simply felt better and that has stayed the same for the last 60 days without the product. I would highly recommend olive leaf extract. It is safe and natural and really quite unbelievable!"   *Janell G.*

Pain Relief

"I have been taking olive leaf extract for approximately one month. I have noticed much less pain and consequently more energy."   *Candy L.*

Joint and Musculoskeletal Problems

"Five years ago I was diagnosed with rheumatoid arthritis. After taking all the medicines I could stand with no real results,

I was informed about some nutritional supplements, one of these was olive leaf extract. After taking it for three weeks, I noticed more flex in my fingers, elbows and neck. There was marked relief of muscle tension surrounding my joints. Overall I am enjoying olive leaf extract with my daily routine."

J.S., California

Yeast Problems

"I have suffered from chronic, repeated vaginal yeast infections now for several years. I have seen several doctors of traditional medicine who have prescribed every prescription medicine available to combat yeast, all to no avail. After less than three weeks of taking olive leaf extract, all symptoms cleared up and have not returned. As a sufferer of herpes simplex II, I would experience outbreaks several times a year. Since I have been taking olive leaf extract, I have had no flare-ups. For me, olive leaf extract is a godsend."

Mary V.

Skin Problems

"I am pleased to say that I have been using the natural herb extract known as olive leaf extract for approximately 60 days now. I have had a recurring chronic scalp infection that modern medical doctors and dermatologists have been unable to eradicate. It had flared up causing very painful eruptions and lesions in my scalp which, over time, have killed quite a few hair follicles. I have suffered with this condition for the last ten plus years, and resolved myself to the fact that there was no help. I am satisfied that I am getting some meaningful results from olive leaf extract. My scalp remains a little tender, but the eruptions have all but ceased. I am continuing to use the product about twice a day, and the skin color is much healthier than it has been in recent history. The results I have gotten from olive leaf extract have been significant because, no matter what drug therapy my doctors have prescribed in the past, none has provided me with the level of relief I am currently experiencing. I plan to continue my use of olive leaf extract, and will gladly recommend it to others suffering chronic skin ailments."

Steven R., California

Skin Problems

"I started taking olive leaf extract, a concentrated natural plant extract. I wanted to see if it would help my psoriasis. While taking olive leaf extract on a regular basis, I noticed that on my upper back, where I had large areas of psoriasis, that now I had just small spots. I will continue the regular use of olive leaf extract and watch for any other improvements in the months to come. I am very pleased with the results as of present and look forward to the continued use of olive leaf extract."   *Robert T.*

Fungus Problems

"I have had mouth fungus for 30 years. All kinds of diets, treatments and regimes were tried to no avail. After taking olive leaf extract, the fungus disappeared within three weeks."   *A.J.R.*

Infections

"I became ill and was diagnosed with a stomach and prostate infection. I was treated with high doses of antibiotics, but never fully recovered. I was troubled with multiple symptoms. Some of which were back and neck pain, fatigue, flu-like symptoms, swollen glands, sinus and digestive problems. I was subsequently diagnosed with fibromyalgia (chronic fatigue syndrome) and the physicians recommended Prozac-type antidepressants and anti-inflammatory drugs, but I refused them. I began taking olive leaf extract along with my regular vitamin and mineral supplements at the rate of one tablet every six hours. After five days I began feeling better. I tried different amounts until I found the optimum amount for me. My overall health has greatly improved and so has my energy and disposition. One very interesting thing has occurred. My finger nails were infected, by whatever infector I had, leaving them wrinkled by sight and touch. Now they are slowly returning to their normal shape. I would highly recommend olive leaf extract to anyone with fibromyalgia (chronic fatigue syndrome.)"

Rick F.

Respiratory Problems

"It was with some skepticism that I began the olive leaf extract program. I have been plagued with a persistent cough and chest congestion for two years. A series of antibiotic prescriptions of various kinds has failed to cure the problem. Imagine my astonishment when, within three weeks of beginning to take the olive leaf extract capsules at the rate of four per day, both my congestion and my cough cleared up. It is still necessary for me to avoid extreme air-conditioning or my cough returns, but only for a brief period because regular use of olive leaf extract seems to be strengthening my immune system and I am optimistic that my problem has finally been solved. I can't thank you enough for introducing me to olive leaf extract." *Dolores F., Nevada*

Flu Problems

"I became ill with the flu, and had several immune boosters, extra vitamins and three antibiotics. My fever was 102-103 every afternoon and this continued even after the antibiotics. I developed paralyzing chest and abdominal pain, being confined to the couch for weeks - not able to hardly walk. My weight dropped to 84 pounds.

Medical tests revealed nothing specifically wrong. I started taking olive leaf extract . Within a few days my temperature started dropping and it is slowly and steadily going down, so that some days I haven't needed to take analgesics to reduce it. The pain is subsiding gradually and my appetite and strength are returning. I praise God for this dramatic break-through and my gratitude is extended to everyone involved in producing this product."

Annalee F., California

Sinus Problems

"I am just entering my third month of taking olive leaf extract capsules, one capsule twice a day. I though you might like to know the following information. I have been a sufferer of sinusitis for many years. Summer or winter makes no difference to me. I have had various antibiotics, inhalants, etc., all of which have provided temporary relief. It always reoccurs. Since taking olive leaf extract I have not had any sign of this chronic infection at all. My sinus is perfectly clear. I also have had mild but painful arthritis in my hands, especially the joints of my thumbs. This has been with me for about ten years. I normally take a regular analgesic twice a day. I had been taking olive leaf extract for six weeks when I realized I had not taken analgesics for nearly two weeks. Amazingly, I have not needed to take any since. In my opinion, olive leaf extract is a miracle. I shall continue taking it as I feel so good, indeed a new woman."

        Renee C., England

Food Poisoning

 "Last fall I ate at a Chinese buffet. Doing so, I contracted bacillus cereus. At first, I thought I was just coming down with the flu. So at the time, I did nothing. Within six hours, I was unable to drive and had to be driven home from where I was. During that time my digestive and respiratory system became dangerously compromised. Luckily my mother knew of olive leaf extract and had it on hand. She gave me some capsules (500 mg). Within 45 minutes, I started noticing a change for the better. Within one hour, I was resting comfortably. Olive Leaf has definitely made a believer out of me. I say that this account of my circumstances is true."

Sam S.

Serious Health Problems

"I'm very ill. The main health problem I'm going to address here is my liver problem. I am turning a dark color and getting weaker. The diagnosis is hepatitis C, for which there is no cure. I had a blood transfusion when I had my youngest child - in '74. There was no screening for this and when my son was about 14 years old, I began a downward spiral which has continued on to the present. I'm told there is no cure. But when I can take amounts of olive leaf extract daily my health begins to mend. I'm a post-polio syndrome survivor and this also begins to improve. I fully believe that if I can get olive Leaf I can walk the earth in perfect health. I say that this account of my circumstances is true and accurate."

Anna S., Texas

Ear Infections

"I have been in constant pain for the last two and a half years with otitis media (ear infection). I have taken three courses of antibiotics prescribed by my doctor, which managed to relieve the symptoms for approximately ten to fourteen days on each occasion, before the infection returned. I had given up hope of finding a remedy for my constant ear pain. I learned of olive leaf extract and have been taking the capsules. My ear infection has at last been helped but I am continuing to take the olive leaf extract capsules in order that my immune system is returned to the correct level of resistance."

James C., England

Ear Infection and Surgery

"Ever since he was born my son had suffered from a chronic disorder in the middle ear, in the form of a build up of fluid and subsequent inflammation/infection. He went from doctor to doctor, and since developing the problem his hearing deteriorated, most probably because of the fluid there. Surgery had been considered on several occasions but this was put off time after time because of the infection. The operation would have meant inserting a drain so that the fluid could freely run out, and it would have left a scar on the eardrum, etc., something which I thought was a drastic step to take. To be honest, I was strongly opposed to my son undergoing surgery, and therefor was considerably relieved when I heard about olive leaf extract gel from an acquaintance. My curiosity was awakened when I heard that this was a completely new natural product. I became even more interested when I learned that sufferers with the same symptoms as my son had become better. Thank you so much for the topical olive Leaf gel. The instructions were simple and involved swabbing the ears with the fluid 3-4 times a day for 14 days. I must admit that I wasn't exactly oozing with optimism, since the doctors had considered surgery on several occasions. One day, my son told me not to speak so loud (I always had to speak to him in a loud voice because of his impaired hearing). I was taken by surprise and thought that I must have sounded quite strict to him. The truth was that after using the gel on my son the inflammation and fluid in his ears had disappeared. The operation that had been scheduled was no longer necessary. In my son's case, the doctors' only recommendation had been surgery. My son's hearing now appears to be quite normal. As a concerned mother, I had been very apprehensive about surgery and had to put off the operation three times. I am now incredibly pleased that I had. I am extremely grateful for the help I received, and I hope this letter will help draw attention to a problem from which a great number of children suffer. If you can benefit from my experience I am willing to offer my assistance so that others can take advantage of and use a product that helped my son. I thank you from the bottom of my heart and wish you all the luck in the future!"   *Line S., Norway*

Serious Skin and Immune System Problems

"Last year I added to an already busy working life by enrolling on a Further Education course. Some of my friends express amazement at how much I manage to do. I work very hard and have had considerably less sleep than I should for over two years now. My personal circumstances also place me under considerable stress at times. Until last year I was always healthy, resistant to disease and fatigue, had excellent digestion and circulation. I was in good shape apart from a bad back due to an old injury. I had some localized eczema which was quite controllable with a messy herbal ointment, and the odd bout of very mild asthma. These were basically allergies, brought on by contact with toxic products such as detergents or cement dust, for example. Last summer I found that my skin was gradually deteriorating, and put it down to the aging process, but by June it was causing considerable discomfort almost everywhere. Then I started to catch colds, had aches and pains, 'pins and needles', indigestion, and the condition of my hair and nails deteriorated. I felt as if I was slowly falling apart. I decided that my immune system was failing. So I started sleeping more, eating more healthily and taking vitamin supplements and cod liver oil tablets. This made no noticeable difference. The skin complaint was kept at bay by using a special bath emollient, wonderful stuff that kept me sane, and

lashings of baby oil. Then under my arms
small patches appeared of extremely painful
eczema, and across my stomach 'scales'
which gradually spread further afield. To
take part in my sport, my way of unwinding,
I had to smear areas of chafing with vaseline
and cover myself in emollient cream to prevent cracking. My skin looked dreadful and
felt so fragile. I could only wear the softest
baggy clothes and elastic was out of the
question. For weeks at a time I was plagued
by colds or any virus that was going around
and it was extremely distressing when I had
so much to do. I was always exhausted and
very stressed. My mother had been using
olive leaf extract and suggested I try it, three
times a day at first. I limited using the gel to
under my arms. It burned at first, so I used
to put vaseline over it once it had dried.
After three days the burning ceased.
Although I did not like the smell or the
colour it left on my clothes this did not matter as the effect was miraculous. It cleared
away dramatically quickly after a very short
period of regular use. That bottle ran out and
I haven't needed it since. I have been taking

olive leaf extract along with other supplements and my health has improved greatly. My skin - wow! The scales disappeared gradually, the burning caused by friction when wearing anything but silk or soft cotton went and it is back to how it was before I started burning the candle at both ends! What a relief, the misery I thought I was going to have to live with has gone. To find a cure for this has been wonderful, particularly as it is coming from within instead of topical application. I was not aware of any 'die-off' effect, but I don't think I'd have noticed it, as I was 'up and down' so much anyway. Since my health improved so dramatically, sometimes I forget to take the tablets as regularly as I ought. I even take them with squash as our water tastes awful. We don't have a purifier and squash is cheaper than mineral water. I usually take two or three once a day as I would forget otherwise. Nonetheless, even though I have not followed the instructions to the letter, my health has remained constant and my skin is fine so long as I remember the emollient which stops it drying during bathing. I don't even need the herbal ointment I used to use. If I feel low I take more. I can honestly say I was extremely skeptical before taking olive leaf extract capsules, there was no 'faith' involved, so the benefit was gained from the product, not my belief in it. This is a real success story for me!"

Alison S., England

Viral and Bacterial Problems

"Feeling quite unwell I decided yet again a visit to the doctors was necessary, hoping this time I would get help. Before I could explain my visit he proceeded to tell me what was wrong, the pains, etc. Sorry he said, but you have a virus and there is nothing I can give you, go home and go to bed, until you feel better. If this rings a bell, then maybe you should carry on and read my story. Although I have another disease which in itself is very debilitating and painful, these very deep pains which are from head to toe are different, and other problems present themselves as well - [health problem], stomach and bowel problems have ended up with me being rushed to the hospital. Laying in bed in such agony that I am unable to get up, feeling so lethargic, loss of interest, unable to stand, etc. I phone a doctor of acupuncture who, over the years, has been able to help. This time however the treatment would not hold. He had seen this once before, so he sent me to see a microbiologist, who examined me and told me I had MRSA. Every symptom of the chronic pain, and many other problems which I had been in the hospital for were due to this. In the 'sixties, I had major surgery. My scar was examined every day to see if it was healing okay. I complained about the intense pain I was in, and was told this was due to the major surgery. I had surgery before but had not felt anything like this. Out of hospital, one week later I was back in, out again, back in again, moved to another hospital, all without an actual prognosis. I was to find that these pains and many differing symptoms, although not quite so severe when I left the hospital, would stay with me forever, or so it seemed. I read about olive leaf extract, and after taking for about two weeks, I had two days of feeling well. It was

a miracle - I could not remember feeling like
this since my surgery. I have had to cut the
capsules back because the die off effect was
great, but I know now what I am going to
feel like once this terrible pathogen has gone
from my body. Every day I feel better than
the day before, after all these years what
more can I say. Thank you."

Sandra H., England

Increased Energy

"I received 60 olive leaf extract capsules over one month ago and I believe it has
been one of the best purchases I have ever
made. I had put in a bad summer suffering
from a re-occurring virus which constantly
made me feel tired and out-of-sorts. Since I
started to take olive leaf extract I have more
energy and feel better about myself. My
doctor thought I suffered from depression or
maybe even chronic fatigue. I feel much
better now and I continue to take at least one
or two olive leaf extract tablets a day. I must
say that they have changed my life and make
me feel on top of the world. What I would
say to anyone is that at least one box is worth

a try. Since I have started to use olive leaf extract I have also convinced my mother and brother to try a box plus I have convinced a work colleague to try it. So far I have no results on these people. I would like to thank you for having sold me this fortunate product and I will be pleased to continue to purchase from your company in the future. Thank you."

Hugh D., England

Viral Infection

"I was diagnosed as having genital herpes in the early 'nineties but I am sure I had suffered from it for a long time without knowing what it was. Stress was the main thing that seemed to bring it on and I tried to simplify my lifestyle as much as possible. I also tried taking several things to strengthen my immune system. Some of the time I felt this was helping until I got over-tired and stressed again. After taking olive leaf extract for a few weeks I noticed I felt less tired and was beginning to actually feel more energy than I had for years. This feeling grew over the months and when I'm clear of herpes I feel better than I have for years. I also notice that the herpes wasn't coming so frequently, and that when it did come, it was usually not as severe. There is an on-going family problem which has given me a lot of extra stress and work for the last year, and I have felt more able physically and mentally to cope with it than I would have done in the past. I feel sure that olive leaf extract has helped me, and will go on helping me to finally get on top of the herpes virus and maybe with other problems as well. I hope this is of help to your team of researchers."

Mrs. E.W.T., England

Hair and Skin Problems Helped

"I have had severe M.E. for over 15 years. In that time I have spent a small fortune on every remedy I thought might help, all to no avail. On reading about olive leaf extract I thought I would have one last try as I'd vowed not to spend any more money on treatments. My hair and skin both are dry and harsh. They have become much softer. I used to wake up in the morning feeling deathly. This has improved. My eyes used to be gritty, heavy, and blurred. They have improved. I feel my muscle and joint pains are easier. My stomach isn't quite so bloated. My tinnitus is more bearable. As you state it isn't a cure, and my energy levels haven't improved so much yet. I do feel anyone with mild to moderate M.E. (C.F.S.) would benefit from giving olive leaf extract a trial. I thought you might like to hear the little improvements which people with mild to moderate M.E. (C.F.S.) are so grateful for."

M.R.

Sinus Problems

"Five and a half years ago I had a dose of sinusitis which was extremely painful and left me with terrific catarrh which has never responded to any antibiotics or sprays which my doctor prescribed. I lost completely my sense of smell and my sense of taste was very much reduced. I had an operation some years ago to straighten the bones in my nose after having had a broken nose for many years and I also had my sinuses washed out, but this was of no benefit at all. The only way I could clear the catarrh was by douching my nose with salt water two or three

times every day. I read about olive leaf
extract in the health food store magazine
about three months ago and decided to give
it a try and the results have been beyond
belief. My catarrh has almost disappeared
and I can smell everything. I was making
my Christmas puddings two weeks ago and
when I opened the carton of spices it was
unbelievable - I haven't had that wonderful
experience of being able to smell those love-
ly spices for many years. I have passed
information to several friends about olive
leaf extract and one of them, who suffers
similarly to myself, has started to take the
capsules so it will be interesting to see how
she reacts. I hope this will be of interest to
you, and many thanks for your help."

Dorothy M., England

Appendix
Olive Leaf Extract's Effectiveness Against Certain Pathogens Invitro

Olive leaf extract has been shown effective against the following viruses, retroviruses, bacterium, parasites, yeasts, protozoans, fungi, molds and other microbes and diseases as demonstrated in laboratory testing including the Paper Disk Bioassay method:

Aspergillus flavus
Aspergillus petrakii
Aspergillus ochraceus Wilhelm
Bacillus cereus
Bacillus subtilus
Corynebacterium michiganese
Coxsackievirus A21
Deoxyribonucleic acid viruses
E. cloacae NRRL B-414
E. Coli
E. tracheiphila
Encephalomyocarditis
Enterobacteraerogenes NRRL B-199
Erwinia carotovora
Geotrichum candidum
Herpesvirus (MRS)
Herpes Simplex Type 2 (genital herpes)
Influenza A

Influenza A/NWS (HONI)
In. A/PR8/34 (HONI)
In. A/FM/1/47 (HONI)
In. A/Ann Arbor/1/57 (HIN2)
In. A/Hong Kong/Richardson/68 (H3N2)
In. B/Lee/40
In. B/Maryland/1/59
L. Brevis 50
Lactobacillus Plantarum
Leuconostoc Mesenteroides
Malariae
Moloney leukemia virus
Moloney sarcoma
Murine leukaemia virus
Rauscher m. leukemia
Newcastle virus
P. Solanacearum
P. lachrymans

Parainfluenza 1 (Sendai) ATCC
Para. 1 (C-35, HA-2)
Para. 1 (Sendai) TUC
Para. 2 (CA, Greer)
Parainfluenza 3
Pediococcus Cerevisiae 39
Plasmodium falciparum
Polio 1
Polio 2
Polio 3
Pseudomonas fluorescens
Pseudomonas Syringae
Pseudorabies virus
Pv. Savastanoi

Rauscher leukemia virus
Reovirus 3 (Deering)
Rhizopus sp.
Rhizoctonia Kuhn
Rhizoctonia solani
Ribonucleic acid viruses
Salmonella Enteritidis
Salmonella typhimurium
Sindbis virus
Staphylococcus Aureus
Vaccinia
Vesicular Stomatitis
Virax
Xanthomonas Vesicatoria [32]

References & Resources

FOOTNOTES

1. Elliott, G., et al., Preliminary safety studies with calcium eleno-late, an antiviral agent, <u>Antimicrobial Agents and Chemotherapy</u>, 1969, 173-176.

2. <u>Nature New Biology</u>, vol. 238, Aug. 30, 1972.

3. Nye, David, M.D., <u>Fibromyalgia -- A Physicians Guide</u>, Aug. 13, 1995.

4. Petroni, A., Inhibition of platelet aggregation and eicosanoid pro-duction by phenolic components of olive oil, <u>Thrombosis Research</u> 78(2):151-60, April 15, 1995.

5. Visioli, F., Oleuropein protects low density lipoprotein from oxi-dation, <u>Life Sciences</u> 55(24):1965-1971, 1994.

6. Petkov, V., Plants and hypotensive, antiatheromatous and coro-narodilatating action., <u>American Journal of Chinese Medicine</u> 7(3):197-236, 1979

7. Perez-Jimenez, F., Lipoprotein concentrations in normolipidemic males consuming oleic acid-rich diets from two different sources: olive oil and oleic acid-rich sunflower oil, <u>American Journal of Clinical Nutrition</u> 62(4):769-75, October 1995.

8. Visioli, F., Low density lipoprotein oxidation is inhibited in vitro by olive oil constituents, <u>Atherosclerosis</u> 117(1):25-32, September 1995.

9. Ruiz-Gutierrez, V., Plasma lipids, erythrocyte membrane lipids and blood pressure of hypertensive women after ingestion of dietary oleic acid from two difference sources, <u>Journal of Hypertension</u> 14:(12):1483-90, Dec. 1996

10. Ribeiro, R., Acute antihypertensive effect in conscious rats pro-duced by some medicinal plants used in the state of Sao Paulo, <u>Journal of Ethnopharmacology</u> 15(3):261-9, March 1986.

11. Zarzuelo, A., Vasodilator effect of olive leaf, <u>Planta Med.</u> 57(5): 417-9, October 1991.

12. Cherif, S., A clinical trial of a titrated olea extract in the treatment of essential arterial hypertension, <u>Belgian Journal of Pharmacology</u> 51(2):69-71, March-April 1996.

13. Ostroff, Steve, U.S. National Center for Infectious Diseases, quoted in "Killer Flu", Kevin Maney and Anita Manning, <u>USA Today</u>, February 4, 1998.

14. <u>Los Angeles Times</u>, August 24, 1995.

15. Tassou, C., Effect of phenolic compounds and oleuropein on the germination of Bacillus cereus T spores, <u>Biotechnology and Applied Biochemistry</u> 13:231-237, April 1991.

16. Tranter, H.S., The effect of the olive phenolic compound, oleuropein, on growth and enterotoxin B production by Staphylococcus aureus, <u>Journal of Applied Bacteriology</u> 74(3):253-259, 1993.

17. Capasso, R., Antibacterial polyphenols from olive oil mill waste waters, <u>Journal of Applied Bacteriology</u> 79(4):393-8, 1995.

18. Mortimer, P., Food poisoning episodes associated with Bacillus Cereus in fried rice, <u>Lancet</u> 1(7865):1043-5, 1974.

19. Tassou, C., Inhibition of Salmonella enteritidis by oleuropein in broth and in a model food system, <u>Letters in Applied Microbiology</u> 20(2):120-4, February 1995.

20. Greer, R. and C. Blau, <u>Olive Oil: the Good Heart Protector</u>, Souvenir Press, London, England, 1995.

21. Rogers, F., <u>Olives: Cooking with Olives and Their Oils</u>, Ten Speed Press, California, 1995.

22. Rosenblum, Mort, <u>Olives: The Life and Lore of a Noble Fruit</u>, North Point Press, New York, 1996.

23. Ewald, Paul, <u>Evolution of Infectious Disease</u>, Oxford University Press, New York, 1994.

24. Richardson, Malcolm and David Warnock, <u>Fungal Infection</u>, Blackwell Science Publishers, Malden, Massachusetts, 1997.

25. Harknett, Philippa, <u>Herpes Simplex</u>, Thorson's Publishing, London, 1994.

26. Ball, A.P., <u>Notes on Infectious Disease</u>, Churchill Livingstone, London, 1982.

27. Timbury, M.C., <u>Notes on Medical Virology</u>, Churchill Livingstone, London, 1983.

28. Crook, Dr. William and Marjorie Jones, <u>The Yeast Connection</u>, Professional Books Publishing, Jackson, TN, 1997.

29. Senerchia, Dorothy, <u>Silent Menace: 20th Century Epidemic - Candidiasis</u>, Strawberry Hill Press, San Francisco, 1990.

30. Stoff, Jesse A., M.D., and Pellegrino, Charles, <u>Chronic Fatigue Syndrome: The Hidden Epidemic</u>, Harper Collins, New York, 1992.

31. Crook, William G., M.D., The Yeast Connection Handbook, Professional Books, Jackson, TN, 1997.

32. All pathogens derived from MEDLINE references contained herein and a Medical Data Bulletin, August, 1995.

33. Garrido-Fernandez, A., Utilization of oleuropein by microorganisms associated with olive fermentations, Canadian Journal of Microbiology, 24(6):680-4, June 1978.

34. Fleming, H.P., Antimicrobial properties of oleuropein and products of its hydrolysis from green olives, Applied Microbiology, 26(5): 777-782, Nov. 1973.

35. Soret, M.G., Antiviral activity of calcium elenolate on parainfluenza infection of hamsters, Antimicrobial Agents and Chemotherapy, :160-166, 1969.

BIBLIOGRAPHY

Fehri, B., Hypotension, hypoglycemia and hypouricemia recorded after repeated administration of aqueous leaf extract of Olea europaea L. Belgian Journal of Pharmacology 49(2):101-8, 1994.

Gourama, H., Mycotoxin production by molds isolated from 'Greek-style' black olives, International Jounral of Food Microbiology 6(1):81-90, 1988.

Health Science Newsletter, Foley, AL, February 1996.

Heinze, J.E., Specificity of the antiviral agent calcium elenolate, Antimicrobial Agents Chemotherapy, 8(4):421-425, 1975.

Hirschman, S.Z., Inactivation of DNA polymerases of Murine Leukaemia viruses by calcium elenolate, Nature New Biology 238 (87):277-279, 1972.

Juven, B., Studies on the antimicrobial activity of olive phenolic compounds Journal of Applied Bacteriology 33:721-32, 1970.

Juven, B., Studies on the mechanism of the antimicrobial action of oleuropein, Journal of Applied Bacteriology, 35(4):559-67, 1972.

MacKellar, F., Structure and chemistry of elenolic acid, Journal of the American Chemical Society 95(21):7155-6, 1973.

Muriana, F.J., Intake of olive oil can modulate the transbilayer movement of human erythrocyte membrane cholesterol, Cellular Molecular Life Science, 53(6):496-500, June 1997.

Petkov, V., Pharmacological analysis of the iridoid oleuropein, Drug Research 22(9): 1476-86, 1972.

Petkov, V., Pharmacological studies on substances of plant origin with coronary dilatating and antiarrhythmic action, Comparative Medicine East & West 6(2): 123-130, 1978.

Prescription for Nutritional Healing, J. Balch & P. Balch, Avery Publishing, NY 1990.

Renis, H.E., In vitro antiviral activity of calcium elenolate, Antimicrobial Agents and Chemotherapy 1969, 167-172.

Visioli, F., Free radical-scavenging properties of olive oil polyphenols, Biochemical Biophysical Research Communications 247(1):60-4, 1998.

Visioli, F., Low density lipoprotein oxidation is inhibited in vitro by olive oil constituents, Atherosclerosis 117(1):25-32, 1995.

Visioli, F., 'Waste waters' from olive oil production are rich in natural antioxidants, Experientia 51(1):32-4, 1995.